TOOTHACHE

A Toothache Manual: Understanding the Signs, Getting Relief, and Maintaining Good Dental Health for Life

CHAD BRUNO

Table of Contents

Introductory

Pain or discomfort felt in or around a tooth is known as a toothache. Tooth decay, cavities, gum disease, tooth infections, broken teeth, and other dental ailments are common culprits. A toothache's pain can be acute, throbbing, or agonizing, and it can range from mild and intermittent to severe and chronic.

• Hot or cold drinks and foods, sugary foods, and even the pressure exerted to a tooth while chewing can all cause pain. If there is an infection present, you may also experience swelling, redness, and fever in addition to the pain in your tooth.

If you get a toothache, you should see a dentist right away so they can diagnose and treat the problem. It's important to see a dentist as soon as possible if you're experiencing tooth pain; otherwise, the situation could worsen. Depending on the core of the problem, a toothache can be treated with a variety of dental procedures, including fillings, root canal therapy, extraction, and more.

CHAPTER ONE
Reasons Why Your Teeth Hurt

Many different dental problems can manifest as a toothache, so it's important to get to the bottom of what's causing it. Toothaches can be brought on by a variety of factors.

• Cavities and other forms of tooth decay are a common cause of tooth pain. Sensitivity and pain can result from a cavity, which forms when bacteria in the mouth produce acids that erode the tooth's enamel.

• Toothaches are often brought on by gum diseases including gingivitis and periodontitis. Inflammation and recession of the gums expose the tooth root, a very sensitive area, and cause pain and discomfort.

• Due to factors such as enamel erosion, exposed dental roots, or worn down enamel, teeth might become sensitive to hot, cold, sweet, or acidic foods and drinks. Tooth pain is one symptom of this sensitivity to certain foods and drinks.

• **Broken or chipped teeth**: The discomfort from biting or chewing might be excruciating if you have a broken or chipped tooth. The pain may come and go but tends to intensify over time.

• When germs invade the soft tissue in and around a tooth, a pocket of pus called an abscess occurs. Extreme discomfort, swelling, and a nasty aftertaste are all possible side effects.

• Wisdom teeth (the third molars) sometimes do not fully erupt through the gums, a condition known as impaction. This may cause localized discomfort, edema, and even infection.

• Pain in the teeth and jaw are common side effects of bruxism, often known as teeth grinding. It usually happens as you sleep, and it can eventually wear down your enamel.

• Adjustments and tightening of orthodontic braces can cause discomfort and toothaches. After a few days, this discomfort usually goes away.

• Sometimes, the discomfort from a sinus infection will be directed to the upper back teeth, making you feel like you have a toothache.

• Toothaches are a common transient side effect of dental operations including fillings and root canals. Tooth pulp inflammation is a common cause of this.

• Occasionally, something uncomfortable or painful can become caught between your teeth or gums.

Keep in mind that these are just some of the potential root causes of toothaches; the exact reason could be different for each individual. If you have a toothache that won't go away, you should see a dentist so that the cause can be determined and you can get the treatment you need. There may be more significant dental complications if a toothache is ignored.

Causes of Different Toothaches

The symptoms of a toothache, as well as the kind and severity of the pain, might vary widely from case to case. Some typical toothache symptoms include:

1. Sharp, Sudden Pain: This sort of pain is commonly related with dental cavities or tooth decay. The sensation of heat or cold, or the taste of sugar, can bring it on.

2. Throbbing Pain: A tooth abscess or dental infection frequently causes throbbing pain. It persists and, in some cases, may even get worse with time.

3. Aching Pain: Aching toothache pain is generally connected with problems like gum disease or the grinding of teeth. It may continue for a long time and spread to nearby areas.

4. Sharp Pain: When a tooth's nerve is irritated or damaged, you may experience a sharp, shooting pain. A quick onset and resolution of such discomfort is possible.

5. Pain that doesn't go away a dull, constant discomfort can be caused by a number of dental conditions, including sensitivity, enamel wear, or gum disease.

6. Pain From Biting or Applying Pressure: A broken or fractured tooth is commonly accompanied with this type of pain.

7. Pain That Pulsates Sharp, stabbing pain may indicate an abscessed tooth or an underlying infection. It has a tendency to be quite powerful and rhythmic.

8. Referred Pain: Pain in one part of the mouth might spread to another, making it difficult to identify the original location of the discomfort. Referred pain describes this phenomenon.

9. Some cases of tooth pain are not constant but rather intermittent. This can be due to a multitude of factors, including early-stage dental disorders.

10. Sometimes the discomfort from a toothache will spread to your ear, jaw, or temple, making what initially seemed like a headache much worse.

It's important to pay attention to the nature and location of the discomfort, since this can help your dentist determine the root of the problem. Whatever the cause of your toothache pain, it's essential that you see a dentist so that you can get the care you need to feel better and keep your teeth healthy. Ignoring a toothache's agony could lead to more serious dental complications in the road.

CHAPTER TWO
Avoiding Painful Abscesses

If you want to avoid the pain and dental issues that come with toothaches, prevention and excellent oral hygiene are crucial. Some advice on how to avoid painful cavities:

1. Regular Dental Check-ups: Visit your dentist for regular check-ups and expert cleanings. Regular checkups and cleanings can help prevent toothaches by detecting and treating dental problems in their early stages.

2. You should brush your teeth at least twice a day with a soft bristled toothbrush and fluoride toothpaste. Don't irritate your gums or erode the enamel on your teeth.

3. Avoid cavities and gum disease by flossing every day to remove food debris and plaque from in between teeth and along the gum line.

4. Use a Mouthwash You can lessen the amount of microorganisms in your mouth and fortify your tooth enamel by using a fluoride or antimicrobial mouthwash.

5. Cut Back on Sugar: Sugary and acidic foods and drinks can lead to tooth decay, so it's best to consume them in moderation. After eating them, you should gargle with water.

6. Water helps keep your mouth moist and clean by flushing out bacteria and food debris as you sip it throughout the day.

7. You can reduce your risk of gum disease and oral cancer by not using any kind of tobacco product, including cigarettes and smokeless tobacco. If you want better dental health, you should try to give up these habits.

8. Protect Your Teeth With a Mouth guard! If you play contact sports or clench and grind your teeth at night, a mouthguard is a must!

9. Eating a diet high in fruits, vegetables, and dairy products can help keep your teeth and gums healthy.

10. To lower the likelihood of dental decay, chewing sugar-free gum, particularly gum containing xylitol, can be beneficial.

11. If you grind your teeth at night, you should talk to your dentist about getting a night guard to prevent further damage to your teeth.

12. Teaching children to maintain a regular routine of healthy dental hygiene should begin at an early age. Make sure they frequently visit the dentist and are good about brushing and flossing.

13. After having dental work done, including fillings or extractions, it's important to take care of yourself as directed by your dentist to avoid any issues.

14. Drinking enough water is important for your teeth and gums because it helps your salivary glands continue to function normally.

15. Stress management is important since anxiety and tension can lead to clenching and grinding of the teeth, which in turn can cause pain in the jaw and teeth. Try some yoga or meditation to calm your nerves.

Toothaches and other dental problems can be avoided or at least alleviated by adhering to these preventative steps and keeping proper oral hygiene. If you do develop a toothache or any oral discomfort, don't delay obtaining professional dental care to address the problem swiftly.

Toothache Remedies You Can Make at Home

While some over-the-counter pain relievers may help with a toothache in the short term, nothing can replace seeing a dentist. A visit to the dentist is in order if your toothache is severe or won't go away. But until you can get to the dentist, maybe these can help:

1. Warm saltwater should be used as a last rinse; to make it, combine half a teaspoon of salt with 8 ounces of warm water. Spit out after 30 seconds of rinsing with this solution. It can also kill microorganisms and relieve inflammation.

2. Pain medications available without a prescription, like ibuprofen and acetaminophen, can help alleviate discomfort and inflammation. Always read and adhere to the label's recommended dosage.

3. Wrap your cheek in a cold compress and hold it there for 15 to 20 minutes. In addition to reducing edema, this can help numb the region.

4. Oil of Cloves: Eugenol, found in clove oil, is naturally analgesic and antimicrobial. You can get some short relief from the discomfort by dipping a cotton ball in clove oil and applying it to the sore spot.

5. Use a cooled (with the tea removed) peppermint tea bag and hold it against the tooth. Peppermint's analgesic effects make it a useful pain reliever.

6. To prepare garlic, simply crush a clove and combine it with a pinch of salt. Put the concoction where it hurts most. Natural antimicrobial and pain-relieving qualities abound in garlic.

7. To make a mouthwash using hydrogen peroxide, combine 3% hydrogen peroxide with 8 ounces of water. Take care not to ingest it. This may help alleviate discomfort and clean the affected area.

8. Swishing with an antiseptic mouthwash like Listerine can help alleviate pain and eliminate bacteria for a short time after use.

9. When pain is the result of tight muscles or a problem with the jaw, a warm, moist compress applied to the outside of the cheek can provide relief.

10. Toothache pain can be alleviated by avoiding foods and drinks that are known to be aggravating triggers.

11. Keep Your Head Up: If you experience discomfort when lying down, elevating your head may help by decreasing blood flow to the painful spot.

Keep in mind that none of these solutions are meant to substitute seeing a dentist regularly. You should see a dentist right away if your toothache lasts more than a few days, gets worse, or is accompanied by other symptoms like swelling or fever.

CHAPTER THREE
Causes of and Solutions for Toothache

There are a wide variety of dental issues that could be causing your toothache, and each one has its own treatment plan.

1. Cavities (tooth decay) in teeth can be fixed by drilling out the decaying area and replacing it with a tooth-colored composite or silver amalgam filling. A crown may be required to restore the tooth's structure in more severe circumstances.

2. Gum disease (both gingivitis and periodontitis) requires expert dental cleanings, scaling and root planning to remove plaque and germs from below the gumline, and, in severe situations, surgical procedures to restore the health of the gums and the supporting bone around the teeth. Good oral hygiene practices, including daily brushing and flossing, are critical for preventing and controlling gum disease.

3. The pus that has built up in a tooth abscess may need to be drained. The infection could be treated with antibiotics. It will also be necessary to treat the underlying cause, which may be anything like tooth decay or gum disease.

4. The use of desensitizing toothpaste, fluoride treatments, or dental sealants to protect exposed root surfaces are all potential therapies for tooth sensitivity. Bonding and fillings are two examples of dental operations that may be required.

5. Teeth that have been cracked or fractured require treatment that takes into account the extent and location of the damage. Dental bonding, a crown, or a root canal and crown may be necessary if the pulp is damaged. In extreme circumstances, extraction may be necessary.

6. Pain, infection, and other complications can be caused by wisdom teeth that become impacted, so they are usually removed. Oral surgeons and dentists are the ones who carry out the treatment.

7. Those who suffer from bruxism (teeth grinding) can find relief by wearing a mouth guard at night. Stress management and relaxation techniques may also be helpful.

8. Adjustments to orthodontic braces can cause temporary discomfort, but this can be mitigated with over-the-counter pain relievers and orthodontic wax to protect the mouth from sharp wires and brackets.

9. Upper back tooth pain can be a symptom of a sinus infection. Antibiotics or other medication for the sinus infection should also help with the tooth pain.

10. Carefully using dental floss, try to remove any foreign object caught between your teeth. Don't poke, prod, or otherwise injure yourself with anything sharp.

11. Inflammation or damage to the nerves inside the tooth can cause pain, and a root canal procedure may be needed to save the tooth by removing the infected or damaged pulp. After having a root canal, a dental crown is typically placed.

It's important to consult a dentist for an accurate diagnosis and appropriate treatment if you have a toothache. Ignoring a toothache can lead to more serious dental problems, so getting it checked out as soon as possible is crucial. Toothaches can be avoided in many cases by practicing good oral hygiene and going in for regular dental checkups.

Dentists and Dental Care

When it comes to people's teeth and gums, dentists and dental specialists perform a wide variety of procedures and treatments. Dental and oral health problems can be identified, prevented, and treated with the help of these techniques.

1. Plaque and tartar (calculated plaque) are removed during routine dental cleanings. This is something a dental hygienist would do to help keep your gums and teeth healthy.

2. Regular dental checkups include a thorough evaluation of the mouth, teeth, gums, and surrounding tissues for signs of oral health problems.

3. Dental X-rays are used to get pictures of your teeth, jaw, and oral tissues. They aid in the diagnosis of cavities, impacted teeth, and bone loss, all of which can be difficult to spot without the aid of a dentist.

4. Dental fillings are used to restore tooth structure that has been decayed away by cavities. After removing infected tissue, dentists fill the tooth with composite resin, amalgam, or porcelain.

5. Dental Crowns: Dental crowns, or caps, are custom-made to fit over damaged or weakened teeth. They bring the tooth back to its original form and function.

6. Infected or inflamed tooth pulp can be treated with root canal therapy. The infected pulp is extracted, the tooth is cleaned, and a filling or crown is placed to prevent further infection.

7. Tooth extractions are performed when a tooth is severely damaged, infected, crowded, or for any other reason that necessitates its removal. Extraction of the wisdom teeth is one of the most frequent dental procedures.

8. Dental bridges can fill in gaps where teeth are missing by permanently attaching replacement teeth to the teeth on either side of the gap. They can make your teeth look and chew better.

9. Dental implants are artificial tooth roots made of titanium that are implanted into the jawbone. They offer a secure and long-lasting solution for tooth replacement by holding in crowns, bridges, or dentures.

10. Orthodontic Treatment: Orthodontic procedures, including braces and clear aligners (e.g., Invisalign), are used to correct misaligned teeth and bite issues.

11. Dentures are removable appliances that can replace a large number of teeth that have been lost. Both full (replacing all teeth) and partial (replacing some teeth) dentures are available.

12. Treatment for gum diseases like gingivitis and periodontitis includes periodontal (gum) procedures like scaling and root planing, flap surgery, and gum grafts.

13. Both in-office and at-home teeth whitening treatments can be used to improve the appearance of discolored or stained teeth.

14. Wisdom teeth removal, jaw surgery, and implant placement are just some of the oral surgical procedures that oral surgeons perform.

15. Sealants, fluoride treatments, and space maintainers are just some of the procedures that pediatric dentists, dentists who focus on the oral health of children, may perform.

16. TMJ Treatment: For temporomandibular joint (TMJ) disorders, treatments may include splints, physical therapy, or medications.

17. Veneers, bonding, and contouring are just a few of the cosmetic dental procedures that can make your teeth and smile look better than ever.

18. Toothaches, broken teeth, and mouth injuries all qualify as dental emergencies that require immediate attention from a dentist.

The goals of dental care are threefold: to preserve oral health, restore dental function, and improve the teeth's and patient's smile's aesthetic appeal. The diagnosis made by a dentist or dental specialist will determine the course of treatment that will be recommended. Many dental problems can be avoided and oral health can be maintained with routine dental checkups and diligent daily brushing and flossing.

CHAPTER FOUR
Exceptions and Cautions

People of advanced age, those with specific medical conditions, or those with other special needs may require individualized approaches to dental care and treatment. Some important exceptions to the rule in dentistry are as follows:

• Pediatric dentists focus solely on treating children's oral health needs. Prevention, education, and catering to children's specific dental needs are high priorities. Dental sealants, fluoride treatments, and orthodontic exams all fall under this category.

- Changes in oral health, like pregnancy gingivitis and dental decay, are common in pregnant women and highlight the importance of continuing routine dental care. Pregnancy can delay or alter the need for some treatments. It's crucial that expectant mothers tell their dentists that they're expecting.

- Patients in their twilight years face a unique set of dental health issues, including but not limited to dry mouth, tooth loss, and gum disease. It may be necessary to take extra measures to deal with these problems and preserve oral health.

Checkups should be scheduled on a regular basis.

• Patients with Medical Impairments Patients with chronic illnesses such as diabetes, cardiovascular disease, or autoimmune disorders may have unique dental requirements. Interactions between medications and infectious disease susceptibility must be considered.

• **Patients with Allergies:** People with allergies to dental materials or latex may need to have their dental operations modified to ensure their safety. It is important for dentists to be aware of these allergies and switch to different materials when necessary.

- Dentists should have the resources and training to treat patients with cognitive or physical impairments. It may be required to modify the environment for these patients in terms of accessibility, communication, and unique approaches.

- Patients with Dental Anxiety or Phobias: Sedation dentistry, relaxation techniques, or behavioral treatment may be helpful for patients with dental anxiety or phobias so that they can obtain the dental care they need.

- Patients with weaker Immune Systems: People with weaker immune systems are more prone to infections. This includes patients receiving cancer therapy and organ transplant recipients. Dentists must take extra efforts to prevent infections during dental operations.

- Patients Taking Blood Thinners People who take blood-thinning drugs may have an increased risk of bleeding during dental operations. Dentists may need to coordinate care with a patient's primary care physician or other healthcare practitioner if they are not familiar with the patient's current medication regimen.

• Medical disorders and drugs can both contribute to the side effect of xerostomia (dry mouth) in patients. Treatments to ease dry mouth symptoms and safeguard against dental decay may be suggested by dentists.

• Dentists may have a role in the treatment of sleep apnea by delivering dental appliances to their patients or by collaborating with sleep specialists.

12. Patients who do not identify with a binary sex system should be

treated with the same sensitivity and respect as their cisgender and gender nonconforming counterparts by dental professionals.

In order to provide appropriate dental care that takes into account individual needs and concerns, it is crucial for patients and dentists to communicate openly about any special considerations or medical conditions.

Taking Care of Your Teeth

Good oral hygiene, a nutritious diet, and routine dental checkups all contribute to optimal dental and overall health. Here are some must-dos for maintaining your smile's health:

1. Brush Your Teeth: Brush your teeth at least twice a day, in the morning and before bedtime. Brush your teeth with a soft-bristled toothbrush and fluoride toothpaste. Don't scrub too harshly or you risk hurting your gums and teeth.

2. Every day, take the time to floss your teeth and under your gums to get rid of food and plaque that can cause cavities and gum disease. Create a routine to check for cavities and treat gum disease every day.

3. Gargle with a mouthwash containing fluoride or antimicrobial agents to kill bacteria, fortify tooth enamel, and mask bad breath.

4. Every three to four months, or sooner if the bristles become frayed, you should replace your toothbrush or toothbrush head. Cleaning your teeth with a worn toothbrush is ineffective.

5. Drink plenty of water throughout the day to keep your body functioning properly and your mouth free of harmful bacteria, plaque, and acid. Having clean teeth and a healthy mouth requires regular use of water.

6. Reduce Your Intake of Sugary and Acidic Foods and Beverages These should be limited because they contribute to tooth decay. After eating them, you should gargle with water.

7. Fruits, vegetables, whole grains, lean proteins, and dairy products should all be staples in your diet for optimal health. Essential nutrients for healthy teeth and gums can be found in these.

8. If you want to keep your teeth and gums healthy, you should stop using tobacco products like cigarettes and chewing tobacco. One of the best things you can do for your teeth and gums is to give up these practices.

9. Wearing a mouthguard can prevent damage to your teeth from occurring if you play contact sports. Use a night guard to protect your teeth from grinding them together at night.

10. **Chew Sugar-Free Gum:** Chewing sugar-free gum can stimulate saliva production, which helps wash away food particles and reduce the risk of tooth decay.

11. Regular Dental Check-ups: Visit your dentist for regular check-ups and expert cleanings. Your dentist will be able to spot developing problems and treat them before they worsen.

12. Consult your dentist about fluoride treatments to fortify tooth enamel and avoid cavities.

13. The pits and fissures of back teeth can be protected from decay with dental sealants, which are thin, protective coatings.

14. If you have crooked teeth or a bad bite, orthodontic treatment can greatly enhance your quality of life.

15. Avoid Stress If you grind your teeth or experience other oral health issues, stress may be a contributing factor. Try some relaxation techniques like deep breathing and mindfulness meditation.

16. Make sure you can afford dental care by enrolling in a dental insurance plan or securing alternative financing.

Never forget that healthy teeth and gums are essential to your total well-being, not simply your appearance. Neglecting oral hygiene can lead to dental problems, which can impair your general health. Maintaining your oral health and achieving a radiant grin is possible with regular brushing, flossing, and visits to the dentist.

CHAPTER FIVE
Improvements in Dental Equipment

Technology advancements in dentistry have resulted in better patient care, more accurate diagnoses, and more effective treatment modalities. Among the most significant developments are:

• Digital radiography eliminates the need for film, produces clear images instantly, and makes X-rays simple to archive and share.

• Intraoral Cameras: Intraoral cameras record high-resolution images of the inside of the mouth, aiding in diagnosis and patient education.

• Dental lasers can be used to diagnose cavities, cure gum disease, and whiten teeth, all while reducing patient discomfort and speeding healing time.

• Cone beam computed tomography (CBCT) scans provide high-resolution, three-dimensional images of the oral cavity and jaw, allowing for more accurate dental implant implantation and orthodontic treatment planning.

• Using CAD/CAM technology, dental restorations such as crowns and veneers can be fabricated in a single appointment, eliminating the need for temporary restorations.

• Access to dental care, even in outlying or impoverished areas, has been expanded through the use of video conferencing technology, or teledentistry.

• Dentistry prosthesis, surgical guides, and models can all be printed on a 3D printer to save time and money in the dentistry industry.

• Instead of using uncomfortable molds, dentists can now use more accurate and patient-friendly digital impressions.

• Dentists can now insert implants and clean patients' teeth with greater precision and less room for error thanks to robotic dentistry.

• **Artificial Intelligence (AI):** AI is utilized for diagnostic reasons, helping discover diseases like cavities and periodontal disease in X-rays and other imaging. It also aids in treatment planning and enhancing patient care.

• **Dental Implants:** Advancements in dental implant materials and technology have increased the success rate and shortened recovery times for implant surgeries.

• Sedative and Anesthesia Techniques: New anesthetic and sedative methods are safer and more effective, improving patient comfort and reducing anxiety.

• **Smart Toothbrushes:** These devices can provide real-time feedback on brushing technique, helping patients maintain correct dental hygiene.

• **Regenerative Dentistry:** Stem cell therapies and tissue engineering techniques are being developed to rebuild damaged dental tissues, potentially removing the need for fillings and other restorative treatments.

• **Biomimetic Dentistry:** This approach focuses on conserving natural tooth form and function, employing materials and techniques that replicate the original tooth as closely as feasible.

• **Oral Cancer Screening Tools:** Advancements in technology have led to better early detection procedures for oral cancers, increasing survival rates.

- **Virtual Reality (VR) Distraction:** VR headsets can help patients relax and minimize anxiety during dental operations.

These technological innovations in dentistry not only promote patient comfort and convenience but also improve the accuracy and effectiveness of dental treatments. Dentists can deliver more complete care, and patients can enjoy more predictable and efficient outcomes. As dental technology continues to evolve, the discipline of dentistry will likely see even more fascinating developments in the future.

Emerging Treatments for Toothaches

While many traditional treatments for toothaches remain helpful, continued research and improvements in dentistry have led to emerging treatments and technology that may give additional alternatives for controlling and preventing toothaches. Some of these emerging treatments include:

1. Laser Therapy: Laser dentistry is currently in use for numerous treatments, but ongoing research investigates its potential for pain management, including treating toothaches. Lasers can help reduce inflammation, sterilize tissues, and promote healing, which may alleviate pain and expedite recovery.

2. Regenerative Dentistry: This area examines strategies to regenerate injured dental tissues, such as dentin and pulp. Regenerative treatments aim to restore teeth afflicted by decay, infection, or injury and may offer alternate answers to standard fillings and root canals.

3. Nanotechnology: Nanoparticles and nanomaterials are being researched for their ability to treat specific dental concerns, such as strengthening enamel, remineralizing teeth, and delivering tailored medication therapies for pain alleviation.

4. Tooth Nerve Regeneration: Researchers are studying techniques to encourage the regeneration of injured tooth nerves to address problems like tooth sensitivity and pain from nerve damage.

5. Stem Cell Therapy: Stem cell research has promise for healing damaged dental tissues and perhaps regenerating teeth, enabling new paths for treating toothaches and related disorders.

6. Microbiome-Based Therapies: Understanding the oral microbiome and its function in oral health is leading to prospective treatments that focus on rebalancing the mouth's microbial ecology to prevent problems that can contribute to toothaches, such as cavities and gum disease.

7. Pain-Relief drugs: Ongoing research into pain management may lead to new drugs and drug delivery technologies that give greater pain relief for dental issues.

8. Telehealth & TeleDentistry: Telehealth technologies are becoming increasingly significant, allowing patients to get remote dental consultations and assistance for treating oral pain, especially in emergencies.

9. **Smart Oral Health Devices:** The development of smart toothbrushes and oral hygiene devices may help avoid dental difficulties that contribute to toothaches by delivering real-time feedback on oral hygiene habits.

10. **Advanced Imaging Techniques:** Cutting-edge imaging technologies, such as MRI and advanced 3D scans, are boosting diagnostic capabilities, which can lead to more accurate and

successful treatment strategies for toothache reasons.

While some developing therapies offer promise, it's crucial to note that they may still be in the experimental or early stages of development, and their widespread adoption in dentistry practice may take some time. Traditional dental treatments and preventive measures remain the foundation of maintaining good oral health and treating toothaches. If you develop a toothache, it's crucial to contact a dentist for an accurate diagnosis and suitable treatment based on current best practices.

Conclusion

toothaches can be a source of substantial discomfort and agony, and they often come from several dental concerns, including tooth decay, gum disease, infections, and more. Preventing toothaches with appropriate oral hygiene practices, a balanced diet, and frequent dental check-ups is vital for maintaining oral health.

When toothaches do occur, it's crucial to seek professional dental care for an accurate diagnosis and suitable treatment. Home remedies may provide temporary relief, but they do not replace the need for expert care. The kind and cause of a toothache might vary, and dentists employ various treatments and procedures to address these difficulties efficiently.

Advancements in dental technology and developing treatments provide intriguing possibilities for the future of dentistry, from laser therapy and regenerative dentistry to nanotechnology and microbiome-based therapies. These developments may lead to more effective pain management and prevention strategies for toothaches.

Remember that maintaining dental health is not just about having a beautiful smile; it is a key component of total well-being. You may avoid future dental issues and enjoy a healthy, pain-free smile by prioritizing your oral health via proper care and routine dentist visits.

THE END